This planner belongs to :

_____

Twenty-three

January

S	M	T	W	T	F	S
1	2	3	4	5	6	7
8	9	10	11	12	13	14
15	16	17	18	19	20	21
22	23	24	25	26	27	28
29	30	31				

February

S	M	T	W	T	F	S
			1	2	3	4
5	6	7	8	9	10	11
12	13	14	15	16	17	18
19	20	21	22	23	24	25
26	27	28				

March

S	M	T	W	T	F	S
			1	2	3	4
5	6	7	8	9	10	11
12	13	14	15	16	17	18
19	20	21	22	23	24	25
26	27	28	29	30	31	

April

S	M	T	W	T	F	S
						1
2	3	4	5	6	7	8
9	10	11	12	13	14	15
16	17	18	19	20	21	22
23	24	25	26	27	28	29
30						

May

S	M	T	W	T	F	S
	1	2	3	4	5	6
7	8	9	10	11	12	13
14	15	16	17	18	19	20
21	22	23	24	25	26	27
28	29	30	31			

June

S	M	T	W	T	F	S
				1	2	3
4	5	6	7	8	9	10
11	12	13	14	15	16	17
18	19	20	21	22	23	24
25	26	27	28	29	30	

July

S	M	T	W	T	F	S
						1
2	3	4	5	6	7	8
9	10	11	12	13	14	15
16	17	18	19	20	21	22
23	24	25	26	27	28	29
30	31					

August

S	M	T	W	T	F	S
		1	2	3	4	5
6	7	8	9	10	11	12
13	14	15	16	17	18	19
20	21	22	23	24	25	26
27	28	29	30	31		

September

S	M	T	W	T	F	S
					1	2
3	4	5	6	7	8	9
10	11	12	13	14	15	16
17	18	19	20	21	22	23
24	25	26	27	28	29	30

October

S	M	T	W	T	F	S
1	2	3	4	5	6	7
8	9	10	11	12	13	14
15	16	17	18	19	20	21
22	23	24	25	26	27	28
29	30	31				

November

S	M	T	W	T	F	S
			1	2	3	4
5	6	7	8	9	10	11
12	13	14	15	16	17	18
19	20	21	22	23	24	25
26	27	28	29	30		

December

S	M	T	W	T	F	S
					1	2
3	4	5	6	7	8	9
10	11	12	13	14	15	16
17	18	19	20	21	22	23
24	25	26	27	28	29	30
31						

Year in Pixels

	J	F	M	A	M	J	J	A	S	O	N	D
1.												
2.												
3.												
4.												
5.												
6.												
7.												
8.												
9.												
10.												
11.												
12.												
13.												
14.												
15.												
16.												
17.												
18.												
19.												
20.												
21.												
22.												
23.												
24.												
25.												
26.												
27.												
28.												
29.												
30.												
31.												

Color Codes

Notes

January

MONDAY	TUESDAY	WEDNESDAY	THURSDAY
2	3	4	5
9	10	11	12
16	17	18	19
23	24	25	26

January

2023

FRIDAY	SATURDAY	SUNDAY	NOTES
		1	○
			○
			○
			○
			○
6	7	8	○
			○
			○
			○
13	14	15	○
			○
			○
			○
			○
20	21	22	○
			○
			○
			○
			○
27	28	29	30 / 31

February 2023

MONDAY	TUESDAY	WEDNESDAY	THURSDAY
		1	2
6	7	8	9
13	14	15	16
20	21	22	23
27	28		

February

FRIDAY	SATURDAY	SUNDAY	NOTES
3	4	5	○
			○
			○
			○
			○
10	11	12	○
			○
			○
			○
			○
17	18	19	○
			○
			○
			○
24	25	26	○
			○
			○
			○
			○
			NOTES

March

MONDAY	TUESDAY	WEDNESDAY	THURSDAY
		1	2
6	7	8	9
13	14	15	16
20	21	22	23
27	28	29	30

March

FRIDAY	SATURDAY	SUNDAY	NOTES
3	4	5	○
			○
			○
			○
			○
10	11	12	○
			○
			○
			○
			○
17	18	19	○
			○
			○
			○
			○
24	25	26	○
			○
			○
			○
			○
31			NOTES

April 2023

MONDAY	TUESDAY	WEDNESDAY	THURSDAY
3	4	5	6
10	11	12	13
17	18	19	20
24	25	26	27

April

FRIDAY	SATURDAY	SUNDAY	NOTES
	1	2	○
			○
			○
			○
			○
7	8	9	○
			○
			○
			○
14	15	16	○
			○
			○
			○
			○
21	22	23	○
			○
			○
			○
			○
28	29	30	NOTES

May

MONDAY	TUESDAY	WEDNESDAY	THURSDAY
1	2	3	4
8	9	10	11
15	16	17	18
22	23	24	25
29	30	31	

May

FRIDAY	SATURDAY	SUNDAY	NOTES
5	6	7	○
			○
			○
			○
			○
12	13	14	○
			○
			○
			○
			○
19	20	21	○
			○
			○
			○
			○
26	27	28	○
			○
			○
			○
			○
			NOTES

June
2023

MONDAY	TUESDAY	WEDNESDAY	THURSDAY
			1
5	6	7	8
12	13	14	15
19	20	21	22
26	27	28	29

June

FRIDAY	SATURDAY	SUNDAY	NOTES
2	3	4	○
			○
			○
			○
			○
9	10	11	○
			○
			○
			○
			○
16	17	18	○
			○
			○
			○
			○
23	24	25	○
			○
			○
			○
			○
30			NOTES

July

MONDAY	TUESDAY	WEDNESDAY	THURSDAY
3	4	5	6
10	11	12	13
17	18	19	20
24	25	26	27

July

2023

FRIDAY	SATURDAY	SUNDAY	NOTES
	1	2	○
			○
			○
			○
			○
7	8	9	○
			○
			○
			○
14	15	16	○
			○
			○
			○
			○
21	22	23	○
			○
			○
			○
			○
28	29	30	31

August

MONDAY	TUESDAY	WEDNESDAY	THURSDAY
	1	2	3
7	8	9	10
14	15	16	17
21	22	23	24
28	29	30	31

August

FRIDAY	SATURDAY	SUNDAY	NOTES
4	5	6	○
			○
			○
			○
			○
11	12	13	○
			○
			○
			○
18	19	20	○
			○
			○
			○
			○
25	26	27	NOTES

September

MONDAY	TUESDAY	WEDNESDAY	THURSDAY
4	5	6	7
11	12	13	14
18	19	20	21
25	26	27	28

September

FRIDAY	SATURDAY	SUNDAY	NOTES
1	2	3	○
			○
			○
			○
			○
8	9	10	○
			○
			○
			○
15	16	17	○
			○
			○
			○
			○
22	23	24	○
			○
			○
			○
			○
29	30		NOTES

October 2023

MONDAY	TUESDAY	WEDNESDAY	THURSDAY
2	3	4	5
9	10	11	12
16	17	18	19
23	24	25	26

October 2023

FRIDAY	SATURDAY	SUNDAY	NOTES
		1	○
			○
			○
			○
			○
6	7	8	○
			○
			○
			○
13	14	15	○
			○
			○
			○
			○
20	21	22	○
			○
			○
			○
			○
27	28	29	30 / 31

November

MONDAY	TUESDAY	WEDNESDAY	THURSDAY
		1	2
6	7	8	9
13	14	15	16
20	21	22	23
27	28	29	30

November 2023

FRIDAY	SATURDAY	SUNDAY	NOTES
3	4	5	○
			○
			○
			○
			○
10	11	12	○
			○
			○
			○
			○
17	18	19	○
			○
			○
			○
24	25	26	○
			○
			○
			○
			○
			NOTES

December

MONDAY	TUESDAY	WEDNESDAY	THURSDAY
4	5	6	7
11	12	13	14
18	19	20	21
25	26	27	28

December

FRIDAY	SATURDAY	SUNDAY	NOTES
1	2	3	○
			○
			○
			○
			○
8	9	10	○
			○
			○
			○
			○
15	16	17	○
			○
			○
			○
22	23	24	○
			○
			○
			○
			○
29	30	31	NOTES

December
2022

01 THURSDAY

○ _____
○ _____
○ _____
○ _____
○ _____
○ _____
○ _____
○ _____

02 FRIDAY

○ _____
○ _____
○ _____
○ _____
○ _____
○ _____
○ _____
○ _____

03 SATURDAY

○ _____
○ _____
○ _____
○ _____
○ _____
○ _____
○ _____
○ _____

04 SUNDAY

○ _____
○ _____
○ _____
○ _____
○ _____

05 MONDAY

○ _____
○ _____
○ _____
○ _____
○ _____
○ _____
○ _____
○ _____

06 TUESDAY

○ _____
○ _____
○ _____
○ _____
○ _____
○ _____
○ _____
○ _____

07 WEDNESDAY

○ _____
○ _____
○ _____
○ _____
○ _____
○ _____
○ _____
○ _____

08 THURSDAY

○ _____
○ _____
○ _____
○ _____
○ _____

December
2022

09 FRIDAY

10 SATURDAY

11 SUNDAY

12 MONDAY

13 TUESDAY

14 WEDNESDAY

15 THURSDAY

16 FRIDAY

December
2022

17 SATURDAY

18 SUNDAY

19 MONDAY

20 TUESDAY

21 WEDNESDAY

○ _____
○ _____
○ _____
○ _____
○ _____
○ _____
○ _____
○ _____

22 THURSDAY

○ _____
○ _____
○ _____
○ _____
○ _____
○ _____
○ _____
○ _____

23 FRIDAY

○ _____
○ _____
○ _____
○ _____
○ _____
○ _____
○ _____
○ _____

24 SATURDAY

○ _____
○ _____
○ _____
○ _____
○ _____

December
2022

25 SUNDAY

26 MONDAY

27 TUESDAY

28 WEDNESDAY

December
2022

29 THURSDAY

○
○
○
○
○
○
○
○

30 FRIDAY

○
○
○
○
○
○
○
○

31 SATURDAY

○
○
○
○
○
○
○
○

NOTES

January 2023

01 SUNDAY

○
○
○
○
○
○
○
○

02 MONDAY

○
○
○
○
○
○
○
○

03 TUESDAY

○
○
○
○
○
○
○
○

04 WEDNESDAY

○
○
○
○
○

05 THURSDAY

○
○
○
○
○
○
○
○

06 FRIDAY

○
○
○
○
○
○
○
○

07 SATURDAY

○
○
○
○
○
○
○
○

08 SUNDAY

○
○
○
○
○

09 MONDAY

○ _____
○ _____
○ _____
○ _____
○ _____
○ _____
○ _____
○ _____

10 TUESDAY

○ _____
○ _____
○ _____
○ _____
○ _____
○ _____
○ _____
○ _____

11 WEDNESDAY

○ _____
○ _____
○ _____
○ _____
○ _____
○ _____
○ _____
○ _____

12 THURSDAY

○ _____
○ _____
○ _____
○ _____
○ _____

13 FRIDAY

14 SATURDAY

15 SUNDAY

16 MONDAY

January
2023

17 TUESDAY

18 WEDNESDAY

19 THURSDAY

20 FRIDAY

21 SATURDAY

- ○
- ○
- ○
- ○
- ○
- ○
- ○
- ○

22 SUNDAY

- ○
- ○
- ○
- ○
- ○
- ○
- ○
- ○

23 MONDAY

- ○
- ○
- ○
- ○
- ○
- ○
- ○
- ○

24 TUESDAY

- ○
- ○
- ○
- ○
- ○

25 WEDNESDAY

○ _____
○ _____
○ _____
○ _____
○ _____
○ _____
○ _____
○ _____

26 THURSDAY

○ _____
○ _____
○ _____
○ _____
○ _____
○ _____
○ _____
○ _____

27 FRIDAY

○ _____
○ _____
○ _____
○ _____
○ _____
○ _____
○ _____
○ _____

28 SATURDAY

○ _____
○ _____
○ _____
○ _____
○ _____

January 2023

29 SUNDAY

○
○
○
○
○
○
○

30 MONDAY

○
○
○
○
○
○
○
○

31 TUESDAY

○
○
○
○
○
○
○
○

NOTES

01 WEDNESDAY
○
○
○
○
○
○
○
○

02 THURSDAY
○
○
○
○
○
○
○
○

03 FRIDAY
○
○
○
○
○
○
○
○

04 SATURDAY
○
○
○
○
○

05 SUNDAY

06 MONDAY

07 TUESDAY

08 WEDNESDAY

09 THURSDAY

10 FRIDAY

11 SATURDAY

12 SUNDAY

13 MONDAY

○
○
○
○
○
○
○
○

14 TUESDAY

○
○
○
○
○
○
○
○

15 WEDNESDAY

○
○
○
○
○
○
○
○

16 THURSDAY

○
○
○
○
○

17 FRIDAY

○ _____
○ _____
○ _____
○ _____
○ _____
○ _____
○ _____
○ _____

18 SATURDAY

○ _____
○ _____
○ _____
○ _____
○ _____
○ _____
○ _____
○ _____

19 SUNDAY

○ _____
○ _____
○ _____
○ _____
○ _____
○ _____
○ _____
○ _____

20 MONDAY

○ _____
○ _____
○ _____
○ _____
○ _____

21 TUESDAY

22 WEDNESDAY

23 THURSDAY

24 FRIDAY

February 2023

25 SATURDAY

26 SUNDAY

27 MONDAY

28 TUESDAY

March 2023

01 WEDNESDAY

02 THURSDAY

03 FRIDAY

04 SATURDAY

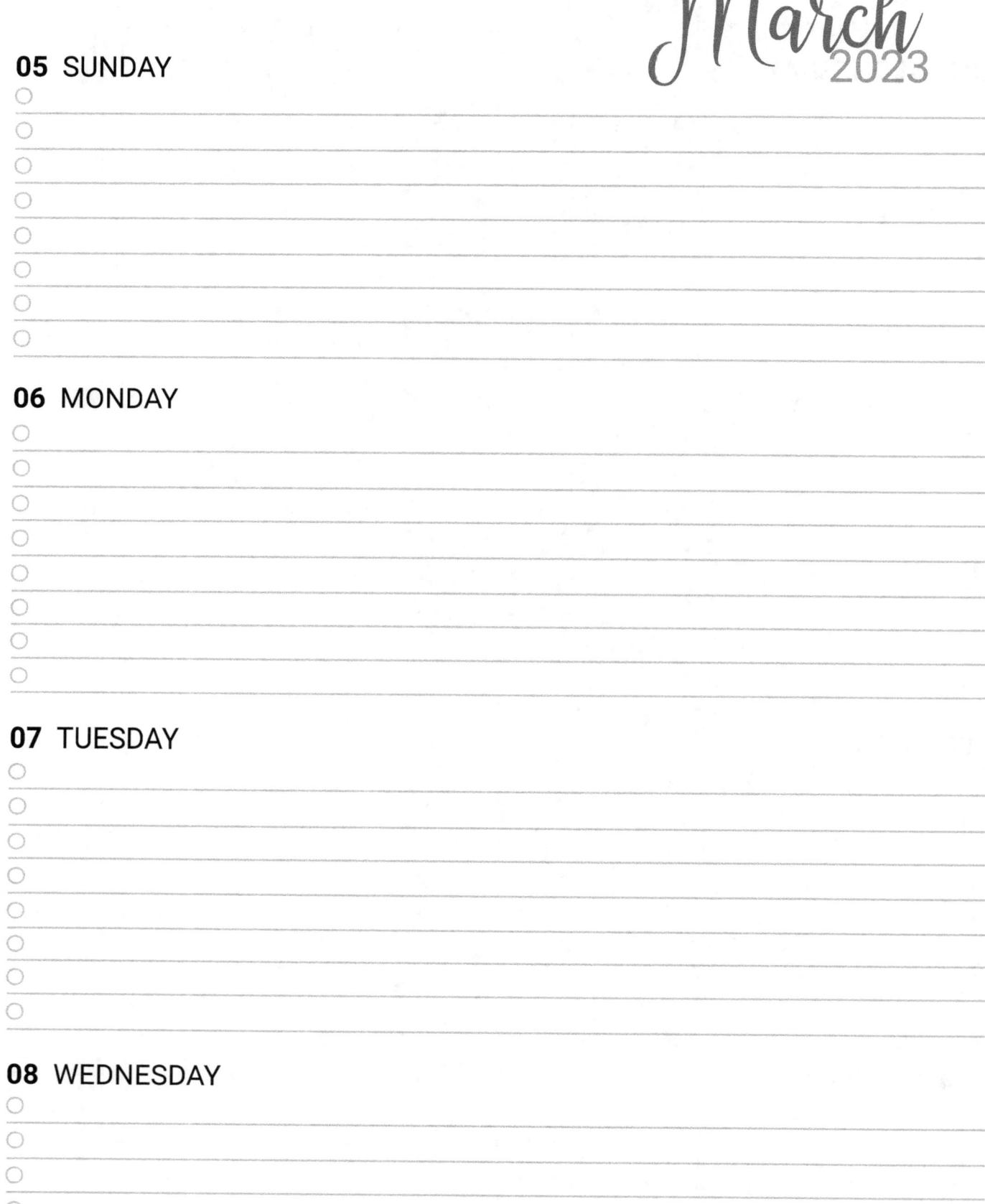

March
2023

05 SUNDAY

06 MONDAY

07 TUESDAY

08 WEDNESDAY

09 THURSDAY
- ○
- ○
- ○
- ○
- ○
- ○
- ○
- ○

10 FRIDAY
- ○
- ○
- ○
- ○
- ○
- ○
- ○
- ○

11 SATURDAY
- ○
- ○
- ○
- ○
- ○
- ○
- ○
- ○

12 SUNDAY
- ○
- ○
- ○
- ○
- ○

13 MONDAY

○
○
○
○
○
○
○
○

14 TUESDAY

○
○
○
○
○
○
○
○

15 WEDNESDAY

○
○
○
○
○
○
○
○

16 THURSDAY

○
○
○
○
○

17 FRIDAY

- ○
- ○
- ○
- ○
- ○
- ○
- ○
- ○

18 SATURDAY

- ○
- ○
- ○
- ○
- ○
- ○
- ○
- ○

19 SUNDAY

- ○
- ○
- ○
- ○
- ○
- ○
- ○
- ○

20 MONDAY

- ○
- ○
- ○
- ○
- ○

21 TUESDAY

22 WEDNESDAY

23 THURSDAY

24 FRIDAY

25 SATURDAY

26 SUNDAY

27 MONDAY

28 TUESDAY

29 WEDNESDAY

○ _____
○ _____
○ _____
○ _____
○ _____
○ _____
○ _____
○ _____

30 THURSDAY

○ _____
○ _____
○ _____
○ _____
○ _____
○ _____
○ _____
○ _____

31 FRIDAY

○ _____
○ _____
○ _____
○ _____
○ _____
○ _____
○ _____
○ _____

NOTES

_____
_____
_____
_____

April 2023

01 SATURDAY

02 SUNDAY

03 MONDAY

04 TUESDAY

April
2023

05 WEDNESDAY

06 THURSDAY

07 FRIDAY

08 SATURDAY

April
2023

09 SUNDAY

○ _____
○ _____
○ _____
○ _____
○ _____
○ _____
○ _____
○ _____

10 MONDAY

○ _____
○ _____
○ _____
○ _____
○ _____
○ _____
○ _____
○ _____

11 TUESDAY

○ _____
○ _____
○ _____
○ _____
○ _____
○ _____
○ _____
○ _____

12 WEDNESDAY

○ _____
○ _____
○ _____
○ _____
○ _____

13 THURSDAY

14 FRIDAY

15 SATURDAY

16 SUNDAY

April
2023

17 MONDAY

18 TUESDAY

19 WEDNESDAY

20 THURSDAY

21 FRIDAY

22 SATURDAY

23 SUNDAY

24 MONDAY

April
2023

25 TUESDAY

○ _____
○ _____
○ _____
○ _____
○ _____
○ _____
○ _____

26 WEDNESDAY

○ _____
○ _____
○ _____
○ _____
○ _____
○ _____
○ _____
○ _____

27 THURSDAY

○ _____
○ _____
○ _____
○ _____
○ _____
○ _____
○ _____
○ _____

28 FRIDAY

○ _____
○ _____
○ _____
○ _____
○ _____

29 SATURDAY

○ _____
○ _____
○ _____
○ _____
○ _____
○ _____
○ _____
○ _____

30 SUNDAY

○ _____
○ _____
○ _____
○ _____
○ _____
○ _____
○ _____
○ _____

NOTES

_____
_____
_____
_____
_____
_____
_____
_____
_____
_____
_____
_____
_____
_____

May
2023

01 MONDAY

02 TUESDAY

03 WEDNESDAY

04 THURSDAY

May
2023

05 FRIDAY

06 SATURDAY

07 SUNDAY

08 MONDAY

May
2023

09 TUESDAY

10 WEDNESDAY

11 THURSDAY

12 FRIDAY

13 SATURDAY

○ _____
○ _____
○ _____
○ _____
○ _____
○ _____
○ _____
○ _____

14 SUNDAY

○ _____
○ _____
○ _____
○ _____
○ _____
○ _____
○ _____
○ _____

15 MONDAY

○ _____
○ _____
○ _____
○ _____
○ _____
○ _____
○ _____
○ _____

16 TUESDAY

○ _____
○ _____
○ _____
○ _____
○ _____

May
2023

17 WEDNESDAY

18 THURSDAY

19 FRIDAY

20 SATURDAY

May
2023

21 SUNDAY

○
○
○
○
○
○
○
○

22 MONDAY

○
○
○
○
○
○
○
○

23 TUESDAY

○
○
○
○
○
○
○
○

24 WEDNESDAY

○
○
○
○
○

25 THURSDAY

○
○
○
○
○
○
○
○

26 FRIDAY

○
○
○
○
○
○
○
○

27 SATURDAY

○
○
○
○
○
○
○
○

28 SUNDAY

○
○
○
○
○

May 2023

29 MONDAY

○ _____
○ _____
○ _____
○ _____
○ _____
○ _____
○ _____
○ _____

30 TUESDAY

○ _____
○ _____
○ _____
○ _____
○ _____
○ _____
○ _____
○ _____

31 WEDNESDAY

○ _____
○ _____
○ _____
○ _____
○ _____
○ _____
○ _____
○ _____

NOTES

_____
_____
_____
_____

June 2023

01 THURSDAY

- ○
- ○
- ○
- ○
- ○
- ○
- ○
- ○

02 FRIDAY

- ○
- ○
- ○
- ○
- ○
- ○
- ○
- ○

03 SATURDAY

- ○
- ○
- ○
- ○
- ○
- ○
- ○
- ○

04 SUNDAY

- ○
- ○
- ○
- ○
- ○

05 MONDAY

○ _____
○ _____
○ _____
○ _____
○ _____
○ _____
○ _____
○ _____

06 TUESDAY

○ _____
○ _____
○ _____
○ _____
○ _____
○ _____
○ _____
○ _____

07 WEDNESDAY

○ _____
○ _____
○ _____
○ _____
○ _____
○ _____
○ _____
○ _____

08 THURSDAY

○ _____
○ _____
○ _____
○ _____
○ _____

09 FRIDAY

○
○
○
○
○
○
○
○

10 SATURDAY

○
○
○
○
○
○
○
○

11 SUNDAY

○
○
○
○
○
○
○
○

12 MONDAY

○
○
○
○
○

13 TUESDAY
○
○
○
○
○
○
○
○

14 WEDNESDAY
○
○
○
○
○
○
○
○

15 THURSDAY
○
○
○
○
○
○
○
○

16 FRIDAY
○
○
○
○
○

17 SATURDAY

18 SUNDAY

19 MONDAY

20 TUESDAY

21 WEDNESDAY

○ _____
○ _____
○ _____
○ _____
○ _____
○ _____
○ _____
○ _____

22 THURSDAY

○ _____
○ _____
○ _____
○ _____
○ _____
○ _____
○ _____
○ _____

23 FRIDAY

○ _____
○ _____
○ _____
○ _____
○ _____
○ _____
○ _____
○ _____

24 SATURDAY

○ _____
○ _____
○ _____
○ _____

25 SUNDAY
○
○
○
○
○
○
○
○

26 MONDAY
○
○
○
○
○
○
○
○
○

27 TUESDAY
○
○
○
○
○
○
○
○

28 WEDNESDAY
○
○
○
○
○

June 2023

29 THURSDAY

- ○
- ○
- ○
- ○
- ○
- ○
- ○
- ○

30 FRIDAY

- ○
- ○
- ○
- ○
- ○
- ○
- ○
- ○

NOTES

July
2023

01 SATURDAY

○ _____
○ _____
○ _____
○ _____
○ _____
○ _____
○ _____
○ _____

02 SUNDAY

○ _____
○ _____
○ _____
○ _____
○ _____
○ _____
○ _____
○ _____

03 MONDAY

○ _____
○ _____
○ _____
○ _____
○ _____
○ _____
○ _____
○ _____

04 TUESDAY

○ _____
○ _____
○ _____
○ _____
○ _____

05 WEDNESDAY

06 THURSDAY

07 FRIDAY

08 SATURDAY

July
2023

09 SUNDAY

○
○
○
○
○
○
○
○

10 MONDAY

○
○
○
○
○
○
○
○

11 TUESDAY

○
○
○
○
○
○
○
○

12 WEDNESDAY

○
○
○
○
○

13 THURSDAY

○
○
○
○
○
○
○
○

14 FRIDAY

○
○
○
○
○
○
○
○

15 SATURDAY

○
○
○
○
○
○
○
○

16 SUNDAY

○
○
○
○
○

17 MONDAY

○
_____
○
_____
○
_____
○
_____
○
_____
○
_____
○
_____
○
_____

18 TUESDAY

○
_____
○
_____
○
_____
○
_____
○
_____
○
_____
○
_____
○
_____

19 WEDNESDAY

○
_____
○
_____
○
_____
○
_____
○
_____
○
_____
○
_____
○
_____

20 THURSDAY

○
_____
○
_____
○
_____
○
_____
○
_____

21 FRIDAY

22 SATURDAY

23 SUNDAY

24 MONDAY

25 TUESDAY
○
○
○
○
○
○
○
○

26 WEDNESDAY
○
○
○
○
○
○
○
○

27 THURSDAY
○
○
○
○
○
○
○
○

28 FRIDAY
○
○
○
○
○

29 SATURDAY

30 SUNDAY

31 MONDAY

NOTES

August
2023

01 TUESDAY

○ _____
○ _____
○ _____
○ _____
○ _____
○ _____
○ _____
○ _____

02 WEDNESDAY

○ _____
○ _____
○ _____
○ _____
○ _____
○ _____
○ _____
○ _____

03 THURSDAY

○ _____
○ _____
○ _____
○ _____
○ _____
○ _____
○ _____
○ _____

04 FRIDAY

○ _____
○ _____
○ _____
○ _____
○ _____

August
2023

05 SATURDAY

06 SUNDAY

07 MONDAY

08 TUESDAY

09 WEDNESDAY

10 THURSDAY

11 FRIDAY

12 SATURDAY

August 2023

13 SUNDAY

14 MONDAY

15 TUESDAY

16 WEDNESDAY

17 THURSDAY

18 FRIDAY

19 SATURDAY

20 SUNDAY

21 MONDAY

○
○
○
○
○
○
○
○

22 TUESDAY

○
○
○
○
○
○
○
○

23 WEDNESDAY

○
○
○
○
○
○
○
○

24 THURSDAY

○
○
○
○
○

August
2023

25 FRIDAY

○
○
○
○
○
○
○
○

26 SATURDAY

○
○
○
○
○
○
○
○
○

27 SUNDAY

○
○
○
○
○
○
○
○

28 MONDAY

○
○
○
○
○

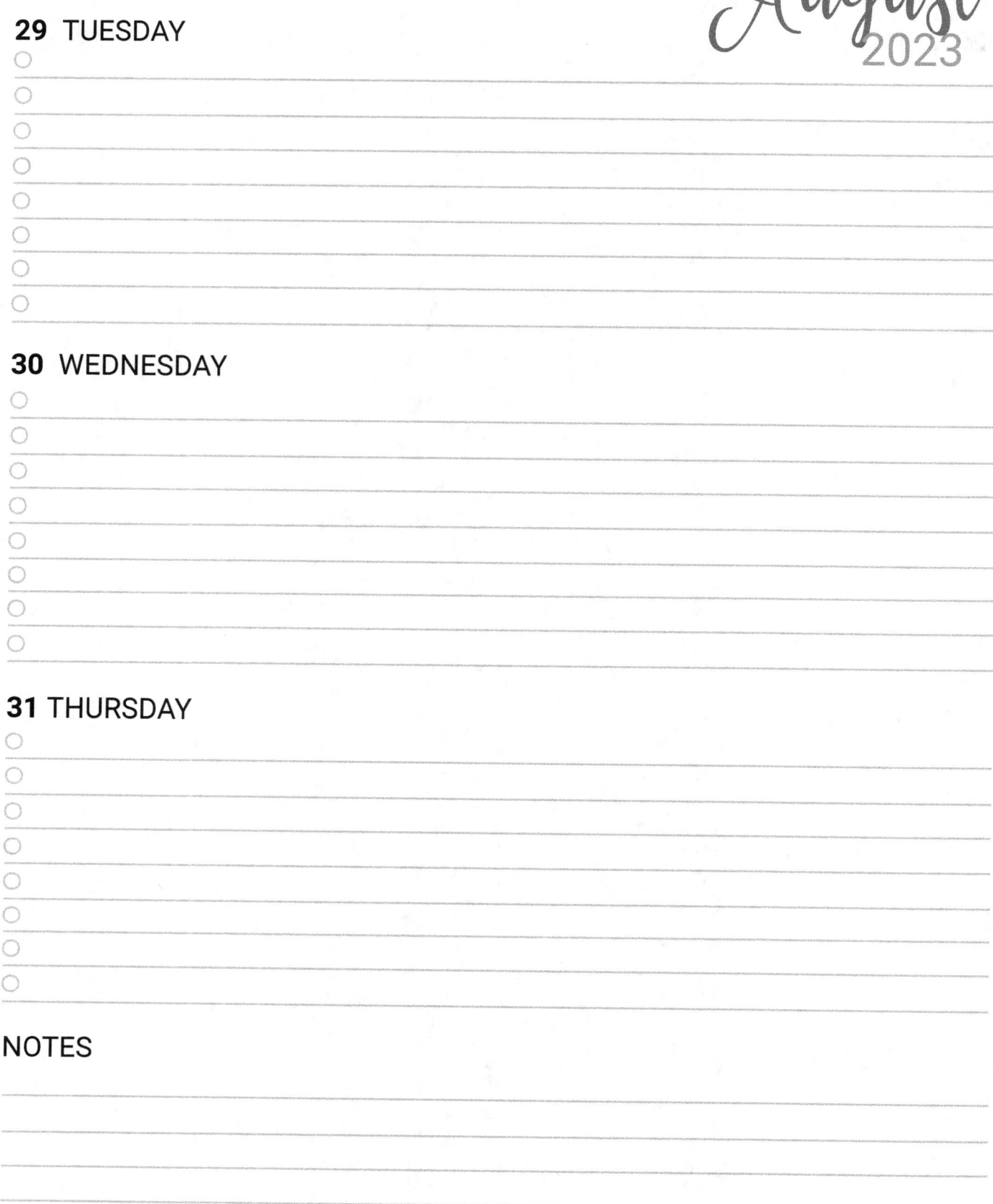

August
2023

29 TUESDAY

30 WEDNESDAY

31 THURSDAY

NOTES

01 FRIDAY

○ _____
○ _____
○ _____
○ _____
○ _____
○ _____
○ _____
○ _____

02 SATURDAY

○ _____
○ _____
○ _____
○ _____
○ _____
○ _____
○ _____
○ _____

03 SUNDAY

○ _____
○ _____
○ _____
○ _____
○ _____
○ _____
○ _____
○ _____

04 MONDAY

○ _____
○ _____
○ _____
○ _____
○ _____

05 TUESDAY

○ _____
○ _____
○ _____
○ _____
○ _____
○ _____
○ _____
○ _____

06 WEDNESDAY

○ _____
○ _____
○ _____
○ _____
○ _____
○ _____
○ _____
○ _____

07 THURSDAY

○ _____
○ _____
○ _____
○ _____
○ _____
○ _____
○ _____
○ _____

08 FRIDAY

○ _____
○ _____
○ _____
○ _____
○ _____

September
2023

09 SATURDAY

○ _____
○ _____
○ _____
○ _____
○ _____
○ _____
○ _____
○ _____

10 SUNDAY

○ _____
○ _____
○ _____
○ _____
○ _____
○ _____
○ _____
○ _____

11 MONDAY

○ _____
○ _____
○ _____
○ _____
○ _____
○ _____
○ _____
○ _____

12 TUESDAY

○ _____
○ _____
○ _____
○ _____
○ _____

13 WEDNESDAY

14 THURSDAY

15 FRIDAY

16 SATURDAY

17 SUNDAY

○ _____
○ _____
○ _____
○ _____
○ _____
○ _____
○ _____
○ _____

18 MONDAY

○ _____
○ _____
○ _____
○ _____
○ _____
○ _____
○ _____
○ _____

19 TUESDAY

○ _____
○ _____
○ _____
○ _____
○ _____
○ _____
○ _____
○ _____

20 WEDNESDAY

○ _____
○ _____
○ _____
○ _____
○ _____

21 THURSDAY

○ _____
○ _____
○ _____
○ _____
○ _____
○ _____
○ _____
○ _____

22 FRIDAY

○ _____
○ _____
○ _____
○ _____
○ _____
○ _____
○ _____
○ _____

23 SATURDAY

○ _____
○ _____
○ _____
○ _____
○ _____
○ _____
○ _____
○ _____

24 SUNDAY

○ _____
○ _____
○ _____
○ _____
○ _____

25 MONDAY

○ _____
○ _____
○ _____
○ _____
○ _____
○ _____
○ _____
○ _____

26 TUESDAY

○ _____
○ _____
○ _____
○ _____
○ _____
○ _____
○ _____
○ _____

27 WEDNESDAY

○ _____
○ _____
○ _____
○ _____
○ _____
○ _____
○ _____
○ _____

28 THURSDAY

○ _____
○ _____
○ _____
○ _____
○ _____

29 FRIDAY

○ _____
○ _____
○ _____
○ _____
○ _____
○ _____
○ _____
○ _____

30 SATURDAY

○ _____
○ _____
○ _____
○ _____
○ _____
○ _____
○ _____
○ _____

NOTES

_____
_____
_____
_____
_____
_____
_____
_____
_____
_____
_____
_____
_____
_____

October
2023

01 SUNDAY

02 MONDAY

03 TUESDAY

04 WEDNESDAY

October
2023

05 THURSDAY

06 FRIDAY

07 SATURDAY

08 SUNDAY

09 MONDAY

10 TUESDAY

11 WEDNESDAY

12 THURSDAY

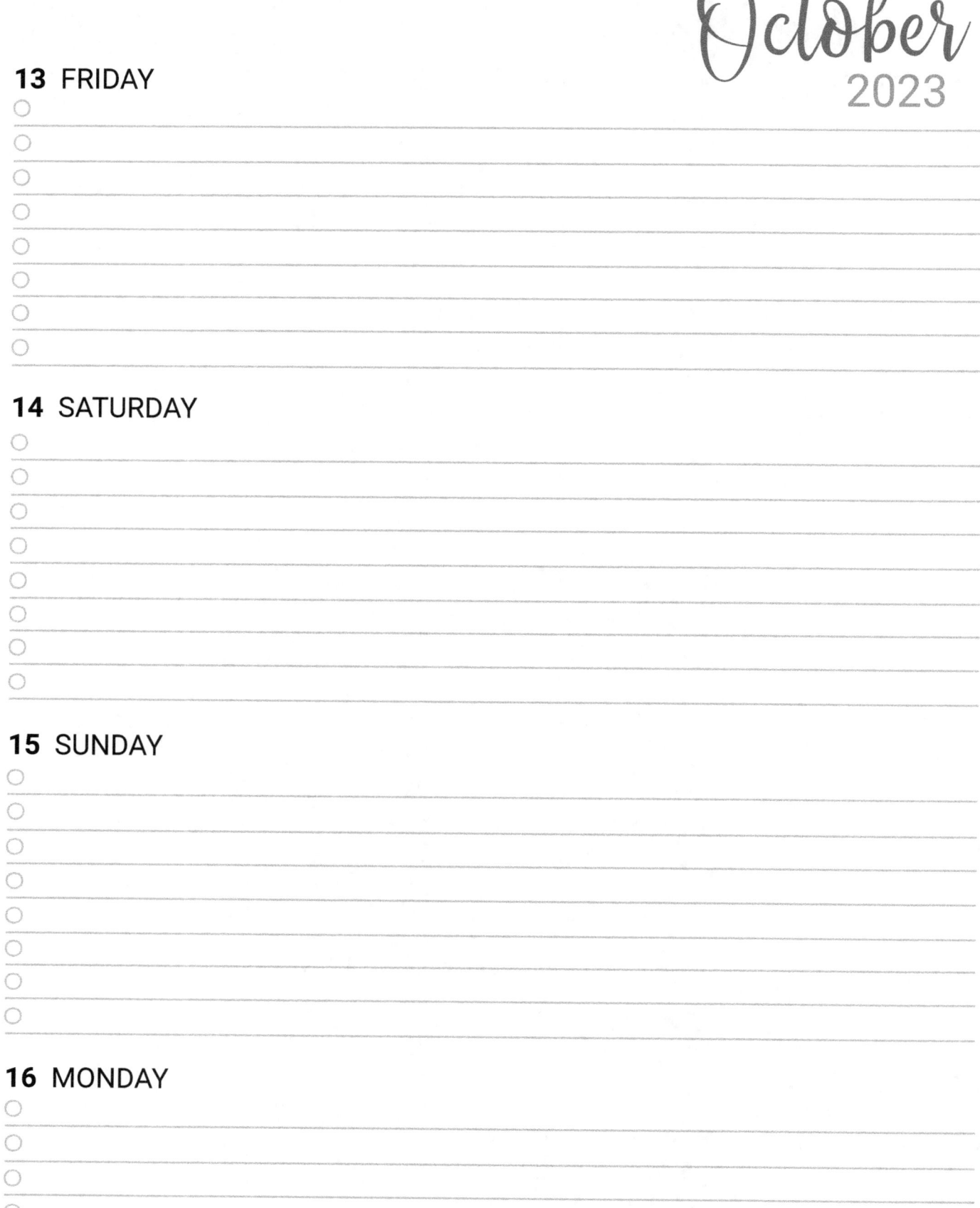

October
2023

13 FRIDAY

14 SATURDAY

15 SUNDAY

16 MONDAY

17 TUESDAY

18 WEDNESDAY

19 THURSDAY

20 FRIDAY

21 SATURDAY

○
○
○
○
○
○
○
○

22 SUNDAY

○
○
○
○
○
○
○
○

23 MONDAY

○
○
○
○
○
○
○
○

24 TUESDAY

○
○
○
○
○

October 2023

25 WEDNESDAY

26 THURSDAY

27 FRIDAY

28 SATURDAY

October
2023

29 SUNDAY

- ○
- ○
- ○
- ○
- ○
- ○
- ○
- ○

30 MONDAY

- ○
- ○
- ○
- ○
- ○
- ○
- ○
- ○

31 TUESDAY

- ○
- ○
- ○
- ○
- ○
- ○
- ○
- ○

NOTES

November
2023

01 WEDNESDAY

02 THURSDAY

03 FRIDAY

04 SATURDAY

November
2023

05 SUNDAY

○ _____
○ _____
○ _____
○ _____
○ _____
○ _____
○ _____
○ _____

06 MONDAY

○ _____
○ _____
○ _____
○ _____
○ _____
○ _____
○ _____
○ _____

07 TUESDAY

○ _____
○ _____
○ _____
○ _____
○ _____
○ _____
○ _____
○ _____

08 WEDNESDAY

○ _____
○ _____
○ _____
○ _____
○ _____

09 THURSDAY

10 FRIDAY

11 SATURDAY

12 SUNDAY

November
2023

13 MONDAY

14 TUESDAY

15 WEDNESDAY

16 THURSDAY

17 FRIDAY

18 SATURDAY

19 SUNDAY

20 MONDAY

21 TUESDAY

22 WEDNESDAY

23 THURSDAY

24 FRIDAY

November
2023

25 SATURDAY

26 SUNDAY

27 MONDAY

28 TUESDAY

29 WEDNESDAY

○ _____
○ _____
○ _____
○ _____
○ _____
○ _____
○ _____
○ _____

30 THURSDAY

○ _____
○ _____
○ _____
○ _____
○ _____
○ _____
○ _____
○ _____

NOTES

_____
_____
_____
_____
_____
_____
_____
_____
_____
_____
_____
_____
_____

December
2023

01 FRIDAY

○ _____
○ _____
○ _____
○ _____
○ _____
○ _____
○ _____
○ _____

02 SATURDAY

○ _____
○ _____
○ _____
○ _____
○ _____
○ _____
○ _____
○ _____

03 SUNDAY

○ _____
○ _____
○ _____
○ _____
○ _____
○ _____
○ _____
○ _____

04 MONDAY

○ _____
○ _____
○ _____
○ _____
○ _____

05 TUESDAY

06 WEDNESDAY

07 THURSDAY

08 FRIDAY

09 SATURDAY

10 SUNDAY

11 MONDAY

12 TUESDAY

December
2023

13 WEDNESDAY

14 THURSDAY

15 FRIDAY

16 SATURDAY

December
2023

17 SUNDAY

○ _____
○ _____
○ _____
○ _____
○ _____
○ _____
○ _____
○ _____

18 MONDAY

○ _____
○ _____
○ _____
○ _____
○ _____
○ _____
○ _____
○ _____

19 TUESDAY

○ _____
○ _____
○ _____
○ _____
○ _____
○ _____
○ _____
○ _____

20 WEDNESDAY

○ _____
○ _____
○ _____
○ _____
○ _____

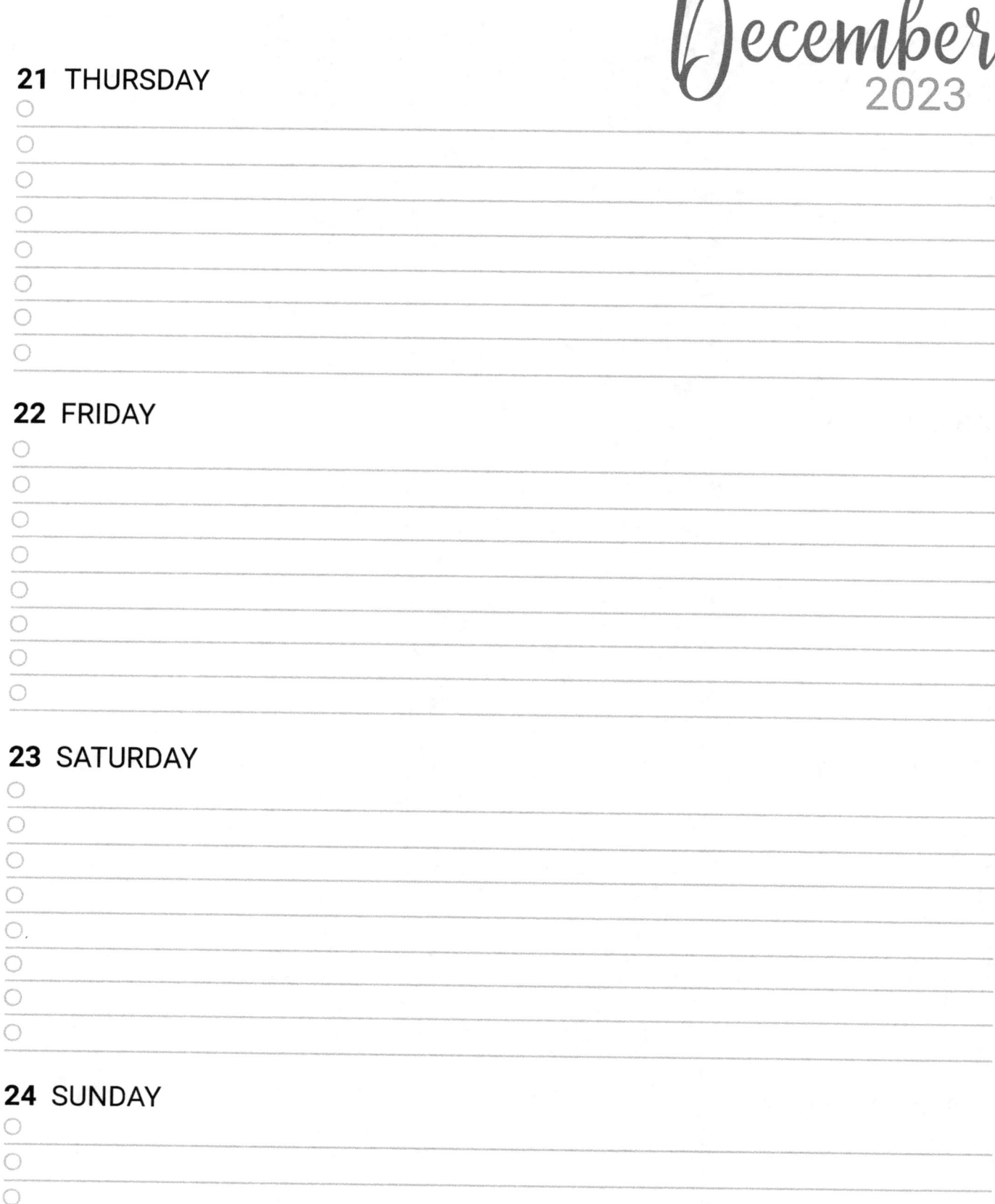

December
2023

21 THURSDAY

22 FRIDAY

23 SATURDAY

24 SUNDAY

December
2023

25 MONDAY
○
○
○
○
○
○
○
○

26 TUESDAY
○
○
○
○
○
○
○
○

27 WEDNESDAY
○
○
○
○
○
○
○
○

28 THURSDAY
○
○
○
○
○

December
2023

29 FRIDAY

30 SATURDAY

31 SUNDAY

NOTES